CW00705063

1 MONTH OF
FREE
READING

at

www.ForgottenBooks.com

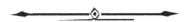

By purchasing this book you are eligible for one month membership to ForgottenBooks.com, giving you unlimited access to our entire collection of over 1,000,000 titles via our web site and mobile apps.

To claim your free month visit:

www.forgottenbooks.com/free1374758

ISBN 978-1-397-32025-4
PIBN 11374758

ADDRESS

DELIVERED BY

THE PRESIDENT

OF THE

Pennsylvania Homœopathic Medical Society,

HUGH PITCAIRN, M.D.,

377

AT THE TWENTY-FOURTH ANNUAL SESSION,

HELD IN PHILADELPHIA.

September 18th, 1888.

ADDRESS.

MEMBERS OF THE HOMŒOPATHIC MEDICAL SOCIETY OF THE
STATE OF PENNSYLVANIA:

Another year, with its successes and failures, its privileges
availed of and its opportunities neglected, has passed into the
account which we must all meet when our life's work has been
accomplished, and we stand before " The Great Physician " who
knows neither school of medicine or sect in the art of healing,
but who, by his own example, commands us to go comfort and
heal by *every* means within our command.

Hahnemann, in his inimitable *Organon*, says: " The physician's highest and only calling is to restore health to the sick."
" The highest aim of healing is the speedy, gentle, and perma-
nent restoration of health, or alleviation of disease in its ENTIRE
extent, in the shortest, most reliable, and safest manner."

Whatever we may credit further of his writings, more than
the law of similars which he gave us, we can all stand firmly
and unitedly on these bases. How well we have this year thus
performed our different duty we may only know here in part,
but cannot know fully ; so it behooves us not to be too hasty
in our conclusions, or too quick in our condemnations ; neither
should we say complacently, " Are not Abana and Pharpar . . . .
better than all the waters of Israel ? " We must familiarize ourselves with, and investigate all things pertaining to therapeutic
science, holding fast only that which is good.

During the year, some who have shared with us these respon-
sible privileges, and according to their opportunities, in their
day, have served humanity well, have been called to their re-
ward, while we are brought together again to utter our experi-

ences, compare notes, and thus be prepared for better results in the year opening upon us. Notably among those who have passed away are:

William M. Zern, M.D., of Philadelphia, September 21st, 1887.

John K. Lee, M.D., of Philadelphia, November 10th, 1887.

Percy O. B. Gause, M.D., Aiken, South Carolina, November 10th, 1887.

Adolph Lippe, of Philadelphia, January 23d, 1888.

I was peculiarly and forcibly impressed with these interrogative sentences of the address of Professor A. R. Thomas, last year, at our Pittsburgh meeting:

"Does homœopathy constitute the whole of therapeutic science?" "Is the physician best prepared to cope with disease in its varied forms whose knowledge and use of drugs is always, and only, confined to their homœopathic use?" "Has the physician discharged his full duty to his patients, in all cases, when he has made the most careful selections of the symptoms in the case?" "May the medical school, in view of its responsibility in the education of physicians, confine its therapeutic teachings to the homœopathic medication alone?" And, without wishing to antagonize the peculiar views of any member of our State Society, I am constrained to affirm negatively to every proposition.

One of the elements that contributed to the phenomenal success of homœopathic practitioners of medicine in the past, has been the fact that, while believing firmly in the fundamental theories enunciated by Hahnemann, yet they were broadminded investigators of truth from every source, and learned in ALL the wisdom of THE SCHOOLS. They were thus twice armed, having a knowledge of what might have been done in each case by practitioners who preceded them; enabled thus to counteract evil from drugging, etc., and, at the same time, having a knowledge of what could be accomplished with better means; while "our friends the enemy" (determined at least in their own minds to be considered such) utterly refused to investigate the bulwark of strength we possess in our "Law of Cure." Indeed, the one thing, in my intercourse with educated allopathic practitioners of medicine in our day, that has most amazed me, has been the utter want of even a slight knowledge of homœo-pathic laws and theories—or, indeed, any therapeutic practice outside of their sect; for surely, if there be a sect in medicine, it is the so-called " Regular" sect.

I come before you to-day, therefore, to plead for greater lati-tude in our own professional intercourse with each other, in all matters doubtful or bearing the semblance of doubt, believing as I do, that the greatest evil in therapeutic medicine in the past has been the adoption of creeds and codes, with ostracism of those who thought for themselves.

What might the " Allopathic sect " not have accomplished in the past hundred years, had they patiently, without prejudice, investigated Hahnemann's discoveries, availing themselves of the truth first formulated by him and his coadjutors. Yea, what suffering and misery might humanity have escaped? Surely, " There are none so blind as they who will not see." I say again, the great evil in the past in medicine, no less than in theology, has been in the adoption of " creeds."

There is something of art and science in medicine, but as in chemistry, botany, astronomy, and all the arts and sciences, there is an ever-widening, expanding, increasing range of dis-covery and improvement. What would be thought of a creed in astronomy with fixed codes? There are laws in medicine, "natural laws," too, which we recognize, as, for instance, the benign law of similars, with others allied thereto, but these are not all there is of law. Rules and principles we recognize, but they are open to change and improvement, as more facts are gathered and generalized. Is there anything absolutely fixed? We may to-day be impressed by a law of nature, supreme in its own sphere, but can we say that there are no other laws in other spheres of the science and art of healing?

We must not, therefore, dogmatize or form creeds, thus sub-jecting ourselves to the ridicule of an intelligent public, but we should hold that all that has preceded in our theories and prac-tices may be altered or amended in accordance with increasing light and the evolutions of general science; *fortunately these have thus far only served to make more luminous and effulgent the fundamental principles of homœopathy.*

It is not to be wondered at that the allopathic school chafe under the effect of the name given us in reproach, on thrusting us out from their sect; it is a good name, a synonym for the words progress and liberality, and we are reminded by "THE WORD" that a good name is rather to be chosen than great riches. The name certainly has brought us patients, and *patience* brings riches and contentment if we grow not weary in well-doing.

The bigotry formerly so commonly manifested toward homœopathy is happily passing away and must do so completely, if we but enlighten the public as to the advantages of its therapeutic results.

Let us hereafter try to sink some of our selfishness for the public good and though we are all busy men, devote at least a small portion of our time to the public enlightenment.

In Pennsylvania, homœopathic practitioners of medicine minister to fully one-fourth of the entire population of the State, who desire to be under our care or desire homœopathic treatment for themselves and their dear ones. *This vast number of citizens are without any representation in the charities of the State*, which is indeed a gross outrage upon us and upon our constituency—and the fact that a sect in medicine has controlled the millions of *money* appropriated from year to year forms an establishment more galling than the church establishment of Great Britain or any other country.

It is for you to discuss how we may enlighten the public and our lawmakers, as to the beneficent laws of our school and attainments of our practitioners as well as to successful therapeutic results, and thus compel proper recognition of our rights. Our motto should be "Equal Taxation, Equal Representation."

For years we have been calmly resolving that there should be an effort made to have one or more of Pennsylvania's State asylums for the insane, placed under homœopathic therapeutic charge, but we never seem to realize the fact that to accomplish this desideratum, we must show the general public the justice or our claim to recognition. The present accommodations for the insane of the State, we learn from the Board of Public Charities, are inadequate, and we believe that the State Executive, as well as many other of our public officials, would favor the placing of a new asylum under the charge of our school, but why should we be compelled to wait such indefinite consummation when our claim is one so manifestly urgent and just?

To this end I have prepared comparative tables showing the results of the treatment in the different insane asylums and institutions of the States of Pennsylvania, Massachusetts, New York, Michigan, etc.,—under allopathic and homœopathic control—as well as other statistical information bearing on the same general subject.

The laws of our Commonwealth, recognizing no establishment in church or sect, should shake off this last remnant of class legislation bequeathed to us by the old world, and compel all those who practice the art of healing to investigate and apply ALL truth available wherever found, especially should it be an effort in our own colleges not to confine our therapeutic teachings to our own school methods only, but avail ourselves of everything known; first, for the cure where possible, and secondly, for the relief, when only this can be obtained for suffering humanity. It is because of the recognition of this divine principle of helpfulness by all means, that we have been enabled to accomplish such wonderful results in private practice and in public institutions.

I herewith present a summary of statistics for the five years ending September 30th, 1887, of the following asylums.

Harrisburg, Pa. (Old School).

Year.	Number Treated.	Died.	Percentage of Deaths.	Number Discharged.	Recovered.	Percentage of Recoveries.
1883	576	39	6.77	139	24	4.16
1884	526	36	6.84	65	23	4.37
1885	564	45	7.97	89	27	4.78
1886	575	50	8.69	64	20	3.47
1887	611	44	7.20	70	31	5.07

Average percentage of deaths for five years, ... 7.49
"   "   recoveries   " 4.37

Norristown, Pa. (Old School).

Year.	Number Treated.	Died.	Percentage of Deaths.	Number Discharged.	Recovered.	Percentage of Recoveries.
1883	1371	123	8.97	238	101	7.36
1884	1366	96	7.	156	92	6.73
1885	1730	125	7.22	185	98	5.66
1886	1847	127	6.87	224	105	5.68
1887	1964	155	7.89	136	76	3.86

Average percentage of deaths for five years, ... 7.59
"   "   recoveries   " 5.85

Danville, Pa. (Old School).

Year.	Number Treated.	Died.	Percentage of Deaths.	Number Discharged.	Recovered.	Percentage of Recoveries.
1883	395	16	4.	52	19	4.81
1884	528	29	5.49	87	37	7.
1885	859	41	4.77	72	41	4.77
1886	996	49	4.91	101	40	4.
1887	1054	52	4.93	208	45	4.26

Average percentage of deaths for five years, ... 4.82
"   "   recoveries   " 4.96

Dixmont, Pa. (Old School).

Year.	Number Treated.	Died.	Percentage of Deaths.	Number Discharged.	Recovered.	Percentage of Recoveries.
1883	661	53	8.	116	33	4.99
1884	687	69	10.	102	28	4.
1885	719	59	8.20	123	66	9.17
1886	742	43	5.79	112	53	7.14
1887	795	77	9.68	118	35	4.40

Average percentage of deaths for five years, ... 8.33
"   "   recoveries   " 5.94

Warren, Pa. (Old School).

Year.	Number Treated.	Died.	Percentage of Deaths.	Number Discharged.	Recovered.	Percentage of Recoveries.
1883	540	34	6.29	83	34	6.29
1884	626	46	7.34	97	36	5.75
1885	782	58	7.41	101	29	3.70
1886	842	65	7.71	119	44	5.22
1887	880	67	7.61	155	51	5.79

Average percentage of deaths for five years, ... 7.27
"   "   recoveries   " 5.35

Summary of Statistics for Five Years ending September 30th, 1887, for Harrisburg, Danville, Dixmont, Norristown, and Warren (Old School).

Year.	Number Treated.	Died.	Percentage of Deaths.	Number Discharged.	Recovered.	Percentage of Recoveries.
1883	3543	265	7.47	622	211	5.95
1884	3733	276	7.39	507	221	5.92
1885	4654	328	7.	576	261	5.60
1886	5002	334	6.67	620	262	5.23
1887	5304	395	7.44	687	238	4.48

Average percentage of deaths for five years, ... 7.19
" " recoveries " 5.43

Utica, Buffalo, and Rochester, New York (Old School).

Year.	Number Treated.	Died.	Percentage of Deaths.	Number Discharged.	Recovered.	Percentage of Recoveries.
1883	2017	131	6.49	776	240	11.89
1884	2187	148	6.76	872	242	11.06
1885	2251	117	5.19	922	247	10.97
1886	2364	122	5.16	964	217	9.17
1887	2367	152	6.42	1014	283	11.91

Average percentage of deaths for five years, ... 6.00
" " recoveries " 11.00

Worcester and Northampton, Mass., Hospitals, and of Taunton and Danvers, Mass., Asylums (Old School).

Year.	Number Treated.	Died.	Percentage of Deaths.	Number Discharged.	Recovered.	Percentage of Recoveries.
1883	3551	240	6.75	1056	231	6.50
1884	3706	248	6.69	1198	259	6.98
1885	3764	247	6.56	1142	265	7.
1886	3945	228	5.77	1395	261	6.61
1887	3804	230	6.04	1318	224	5.88

Average percentage of deaths for five years, ... 6.36
" " recoveries " 6.59

Middletown, New York (Homœopathic).

Year.	Number Treated.	Died.	Percentage of Deaths.	Number Discharged.	Recovered.	Percentage of Recoveries.
1883	410	18	4.39	150	69	16.82
1884	423	21	4.96	141	68	16.07
1885	486	27	5.55	131	66	13.58
1886	568	17	2.99	157	80	14.08
1887	642	22	3.42	187	96	14.95

Average percentage of deaths for five years, ... 4.26
" " recoveries " 15.10

Westborough, Mass. (Homœopathic).

Year.	Number Treated.	Died.	Percentage of Deaths.	Number Discharged.	Recovered.	Percentage of Recoveries.
1887	430	19	4.4	123	55	12.79

Average percentage of deaths, ... 4.4
" " recoveries, ... 12.79

I append also the following extract from the report of the Massachusetts State Board of Charities for the year 1887, the percentage of recoveries and the word homœopathic, after Westborough Hospital, being added by me :

[FROM REPORT OF STATE BOARD OF CHARITIES FOR 1887.]

"Among the 530 patients who have been admitted at Westborough in the past thirteen months nearly half have been transferred from the older hospitals, and more than two-thirds were chronic cases. . . . . Notwithstanding this fact the recoveries have been considerable, and the current cost no greater than it was natural to estimate for a new hospital managed by persons who had *not* before directed such an establishment.

" The Westborough Hospital has met with many difficulties in its first year, arising in part from the defective work done in fitting up the basement of the old school buildings, which have been made over into a very serviceable hospital, and partly from the inexperience of the managers, natural to a new establish-

ment. The accidental introduction of diphtheria and its propagation (in some way not yet fully understood) increased those
· difficulties; but an examination of its results at the end of the present calendar year will probably show that it has been as successful as new hospitals usually are; and in some respects its record is very gratifying. The death-rate among its patients has been considerably less than that of most hospitals in the State, and even less than the death-rate at the Bridgewater Asylum, the patients for which were generally selected because of their good state of health, while the Westborough patients, in part, had been newly committed, and, therefore, were more likely to die in their first year than those removed from other hospitals. The figures of the death-rate, brought to the same standard of comparison, are approximately as follows, arranged in order downward from the highest to the lowest:

Hospitals.	Whole No.	Deaths.	Death rate.	Percentage of Recoveries.
Worcester Asylum	444	38	8.5.	....
Tewksbury Asylum	442	33	7.4	....
Boston Hospital	330	22	6.7	....
Danvers Hospital	1188	79	6.6	5.4
Taunton Hospital	934	39	6.3	6.3
Worcester Hospital	1057	61	5.8	7.
Bridgewater Asylum	155	8	5.1	....
Northampton Hospital	633	31	4.9	4.2
Westborough Hospital (Homœopathic)	517	25*	4.8½	12.79

" The Westborough figures are the actual numbers for fifty-two weeks, instead of the forty-two weeks between December 7th and October 1st. The new hospital is lowest on the list, and has a death-rate but little more than three-fourths as great as that of the eight institutions above mentioned, when taken together, with their whole number of patients reduced to the actual aggregate of different persons therein residing during the year. This is a favorable showing, and it is to be hoped, though hardly expected, that the same low death-rate will be maintained in subsequent years."*

* Let it be remembered that the above facts are part of the report of the Massachusetts State Board, and not my words.

The following is a summary of the statistics for twenty-one months, from September 30th, 1886, to June 30th, 1888 (the Legislature having changed the end of the fiscal year from September 30th to June 30th) of the Asylum at Ionia, Michigan (Homœopathic).

Number of patients remaining September 30th, 1886, . . 95 .
Number of patients admitted during period to June 30th, 1888, 47

Total number treated, ... 142

Number of recoveries during period, ... 17
Per cent. of recoveries during period on whole number, . . 12
Per cent. of deaths for 12 months ending Sept. 30th, 1887, . 2⅗
Per cent. of deaths for 9 months ending June 30th, 1888, . 3⅗

Most of these patients were chronics, hence the seeming low per cent. of cures, but the per cent. of cures of patients admitted during the period was 36 per cent.

DEDUCTIONS.

The percentage of deaths under old-school treatment in Pennsylvania as compared with old-school treatment in New York is one-seventh higher, while the percentage of recoveries in the five years is only one-half Why so great a difference, if not because of the stimulating influence of the one homœopathic asylum at Middletown? *and why, in the name of humanity, should this large number of unfortunates be allowed to suffer on worse than death indefinitely, if even old-school treatment in New York could give the required help?*

But when we come to compare homœopathic supervision elsewhere with Pennsylvania institutions the contrast is simply amazing:

The percentage of deaths under allopathic treatment in Pennsylvania, ... 7.19
Middletown, New York (Homœopathic), ... 4.26
Westborough, Mass. (Homœopathic), ... 4.8*
Ionia, Michigan (Homœopathic), ... 2⅗ to 3⅗

The percentage of recoveries under allopathic treatment in Pennsylvania shows the outrageously low average of almost *nil.*

---

* Actually 4.4.

(about five per cent.), while we have the wonderful record under homœopathic treatment at—

Middletown, New York, ...	15.10 per cent.
Westborough, Mass., ...	12.79 "
Ionia, Michigan, ...	12.00 "
" " Patients admitted during year, .	36.00 "

With such results, which school of medicine should be taunted with "*vis medicatrix naturæ?*" HOW MANY DID KINDLY NATURE CURE?—five per cent.? Surely our enlightened and humane lawmakers can no longer close their eyes to such figures—the naked statistics furnished by those who have in the past been in no way desirous of helping the cause of homœopathy.

The State Board of Charities of Massachusetts admit (see part of their report above):

First. That our treatment could not show its best results because of an epidemic of diphtheria, defective plumbing, etc., and the large number of chronic cases shoved on the institution. The question naturally arises, what would have been the decrease in the death-rate, as well as increase in percentage of recoveries, had the treatment been untrammelled.

With regard to the Middletown Homœopathic Insane Asylum the same fact obtains—incurable chronic cases, not only from the other institutions of the State, *their worst cases*, but as well from Pennsylvania (for where is there a prominent homœopathic physician in this State who has not sent a patient to Middletown for homœopathic treatment, being unable to secure such in our own State).

Allowance should, therefore, be made for these facts, which demonstrate that the homœopathic practice will, under favorable circumstances, cure four to one as compared with the treatment at present received in the old-school "*Insane hospitals*" of Pennsylvania. But these are not "Insane hospitals;" rather should they be christened "Houses of restraint," where the inmates are herded together awaiting only death or "*vis medicatrix naturæ.*" Think of it! Only five out of every hundred insane persons may hope for cure. *Is there any science in old school medicine in Pennsylvania?*

There is also an economic side to this question of the treatment of the State's insane. In the treatment of other diseases there is the same or greater proportion of cases. Take the well-established test treatment of pneumonia. According to the records, the mortality was:

Under allopathic treatment, ... 20.5 per cent.
 " non-interference treatment, ... 7.4 "
 " homœopathic " . . . . 6 "

But this is not all. The duration of the disease was:

Under allopathic treatment, ... 31 days
 " non-interference treatment, ... 28 "
 " homœopathic " . . . . . 12 "

What would be the saving to the State of Pennsylvania for labor, hospital, and other expenses in public institutions with a change of management?

The following summary of statistics is from the Michigan State Prison. This prison has been changed several times from one school to the other. I give first three years under allopathic care, then three years under homœopathic care. The prison passed back into allopathic hands, and I give two years under allopathic care, followed by two years under homœopathic care:

	Average No. of Convicts per annum.	Total No. of deaths.	Total No. days labor lost.	Total Cost of Hospital stores.
Allopathic care, 3 years.	435	39	23,000	$1678.00
Homœopathic care, 3 years	545	20	10,000	500.00
Allopathic, 2 years . .	Not known.	Not known	24,000	1800.00
Homœopathic 2 years .	Not known.	Not known	11,000	900.00

I regret that I cannot give other figures I have seen in print, which, I think, would fully demonstrate *the fact* that half the total number of days' labor lost in State institutions, due to sickness, might be saved, at a reduced expense to one-third the present outlay for hospital stores, care, etc.

In the five years represented by the figures above given, the population of the insane hospitals of Pennsylvania has increased from thirty-five hundred to fifty-three hundred, a total increase of eighteen hundred, or one-third. At the same ratio of increase what will be done with these poor, unfortunate creatures five years hence? *The almshouses of the different counties are already overcrowded* with them, and these latter without even the shadow of medical supervision supposed to be given in so-called " Insane asylums."

It seems to me that, if each member of our State Society would properly present even these meagre statistics, with others at their command, to their constituencies and members of the Legislature, arousing indignation at the outrageous ostracism by " *the powers that be* " of so respectable a portion of taxpayers, it would not be many months until insane asylums, and appropriations for hospitals in general, would be more equitably administered.

I would suggest the appointment of a bureau for the collection, collation, and promulgation of statistics from every source available, showing comparison of treatment, and that, if possible, a fund be secured to this end. We need not fear comparison. The old school have no figures with which they can meet those already in our possession.

It is a satisfaction to be able to report a general advance of our school throughout the State, and *yet there is room.* The field, already overcrowded by old-school practitioners, is only partly occupied by us. Not only in our own State, but everywhere, our cause is moving steadily forward in the improvement and establishing of hospitals, and the occupation of outlying districts by thoroughly educated and efficient PHYSICIANS, not Sectarians, who crowd out the old-school methods and practitioners with their antiquated procedures, causing an increase of the longevity of the race. How much of the marked increase in longevity of the present generation may be traced principally to the teachings and practice of homœopathy is an intensely interesting question?

It is also gratifying to be able to state that all homœopathic colleges east of the Ohio river require a three-years' course of *college* study before graduation is permitted, and that the American Institute of Homœopathy at its last meeting adopted a resolution requiring all the homœopathic colleges in the United States to adopt the three-years' course not later than 1891.

Very few of the allopathic colleges do more than *recommena* a three-years' course of college study.

Papers and Discussions.

Many papers of our State Society, prepared by our members at great expenditure of time and strength, in my estimation, do not accomplish the good justified by the outlay because of delay and method of publication. I would urge upon you the desirability of some action similar to that lately taken by the American Institute of Homœopathy, to allow of their publication whenever desirable in the current literature of homœopathy, under certain restrictions. This society owes it to its general excellence, it being acknowledged as one of the best of our State societies, and should, therefore, take the lead of other societies in this direction for the general good.

I would require:

First. That all papers to be published outside of the TRANSACTIONS shall be furnished in duplicate, and *only* secured through the Secretary of the State Society.

Secondly. Restriction of number of papers furnished to any one periodical to be two or less.

Thirdly. We might stipulate with each journal that publishes our papers that they shall carry an advertisement of one page, announcing the Table of Contents of our Society TRANSACTIONS, etc.

I would urge upon you the desirability of the discussion of each subject brought before our meeting, and for the sake of accuracy, etc., where remedies are mentioned, the potency used be always specified.

Time and Place of Meeting.

It has been suggested that probably a change of the time of the meeting of this society to spring instead of fall, so as to take advantage of the time of meeting of the alumni associations and commencement exercises of colleges might prove advantageous in securing a larger attendance. I would advise a thorough consideration of this matter.

Ladies and gentlemen, allow me again to express to you my sincere thanks for the honor you conferred in electing me, so young a member of this Society, to preside at this time. I can only crave your indulgence if I should unintentionally err in fulfilling the duties of the office, and wish for each of you a very pleasant sojourn in Philadelphia, and a profitable session of the Society.

APPENDIX.

HOMŒOPATHS AND ALLOPATHS AT THE BAR OF STATUTES.

" Twenty-six Years of the NEW THERAPEUTICS *at the Five Points."*

TREATMENT of typhus fever at Five Points Homœopathic Mission Hospital, New York, during epidemics, 1861 to 1871, 285 cases, with only 2 deaths. This record is most remarkable when it is considered that Murcheson's statistics for 23 years at the London Fever Hospital shows a mortality of 18.92 per cent.

Forty-five cases of gangrene of the mouth; 2 deaths. 75 per cent. is given as a low mortality rate under old-school treatment. (See J. Solis Cohen, in Pepper's " System of Medicine.")

Pure homœopathic treatment of the diarrhœal diseases has been very effectual at the House of Industry, notwithstanding its situation in the heart of a region so overcrowded and filthy that for many years it has borne the name of the most unsanitary part of New York city, and where even now the little victims of " summer complaint " die by hundreds during the heated term of every year. During the cholera epidemic of 1866, by the most scrupulous cleanliness and careful attention to diet, and by treatment of all cases of diarrhœa at their inception, the institution was enabled to report but one death among its 200 inmates, though it had an unpaved street in front, filled with garbage, and was surrounded by tumble-down tenements, inhabited by the most degraded and filthy beings in the city, among whom cholera claimed its victims by the score. The records show 33 cases of enteritis, 91 of dysentery, 25 of cholera morbus, 6 of cholera infantum, and 1164 of diarrhœa—1319 cases in all, with 4 deaths: 3 from cholera infantum, and 1 from dysentery.

The old familiar remedies first used by Samuel Hahnemann for croup have proved their power over that destroyer of childhood, at the Five Points, as they have wherever they have been given a trial. The experience of the institution tends to corroborate the belief which is held by many members of this society, that many cases which would otherwise develop into true croup may, in the majority of instances, be arrested by homœopathic treatment in the primary stage of acute catarrhal laryngitis before the croupous exudation takes place. Beginning, laryngitis has been treated wholesale in the dormitories with good effect, and only the more serious case have been entered into the records. Ninety-nine cases of croup, spasmodic and membranous, have been treated during the 26 years, and 8 have proved fatal.

During these 26 years *Belladonna* has been given as a prophylactic to all the children in the House at every outbreak of scarlet fever, with an effect in limiting contagion, even from cases of the most malignant type, which has seemed very evident to the physician in charge. Some 150 children from the tenements in Baxter, Mott, and Mulberry streets, which are the *bete noir* of the New York Health Board, mix daily in the school with the House children, bringing with them every variety of disease that can be communicated from one child to another, so that our records of 88 cases of scarlatina for this period shows a remarkable immunity, in view of the readiness with which the scarlatinal germ, especially, is conveyed in the clothing, etc., of brothers, sisters, or neighbors, and the length of time through which its activity is often retained. Three of these 88 cases died.

Smallpox has not appeared in the House since March, 1864, with the exception of one case in 1881.

Only 3 of the 84 cases of typhoid fever proved fatal, and 28 cases of relapsing fever, 8 cases of varioloid, 3 cases of malignant pustule, 114 cases of erysipelas, and 171 cases of whooping cough have been treated without a death.

Other extracts from these statistics which seem worthy of notice are, 74 cases of diphtheria, with 10 deaths; 601 cases of measles, with 10 deaths; 179 cases of croupous pneumonia, with 4 deaths; 7 cases of typhoid pneumonia, with 1 death; 36 cases of catarrhal pneumonia, with 2 deaths; 19 cases of capillary bronchitis, with 5 deaths; 33 cases of Bright's disease, with 6 deaths; and 11 cases of cerebro-spinal meningitis, with 3 deaths.

Opium, Chloral, Morphia, and the *Bromides,* with the various emetics, purgatives and tonics, whose use is characteristic of old-school practice, have not since 1861 been given to the children at the House of Industry. These children are largely of the most unfavorable class, full of scrofula, syphilis, and all manner of inherited predisposition to disease, andthey live in a part of New York city probably the least desirable from a sanitary point of view. They have been treated in accordance with the law of similars—by that therapeutic method which is called the homœopathic. The results shown by this table, from which I have quoted, will bear comparison with those obtained in any institution or hospital for children, wherever located, and they would hardly be considered discreditable to any mode of treatment by physicians of any school.

In the history of this institution from January 14th, 1861 to October 1st, 1887, under homœopathic medication, there was a total of 25,552 patients of all classes of diseases, the subjects being of the lowest strata of the population of New York city, and yet there were but 158 deaths—less than 1 per cent.—*North American Journal of Homœopathy,* June, 1888.

EXTRACT FROM REPORT OF THE WARD'S ISLAND HOSPITAL, HOMŒOPATHIC, 1887.

This hospital is now in its thirteenth year, and has, since its opening in 1875, a daily average of 531 patients, with a mortality of 5.6 per cent.

SUMMARY FOR NINE MONTHS, JAN. 1ST TO SEPT. 30TH, 1887.

Bellevue (Allopathic), 7337 cases, with 700 deaths, or 9.0 per cent. mortality.
Charity,   "   5330   "   411   "   7.7   "   "
Homœopathic,   3068   "   202   "   6.5   "   "

Referring to the report of 1882, we find that Belevue treated 9709 patients, with a mortality of 1235, or 12.72 per cent. In the table of the causes of death we find the following percentages : Phthisis, 21.45; pneumonia, 11 ; nephritis, 7.6; alcoholism, 6 ; typhoid fever, 2.26 ; erysipelas, 2 ; injuries, 12.22.

The daily per capita cost was 49 cents. The daily cost for drugs and liquors was 6.54 cents.

Charity Hospital treated 8200 patients, with a death-rate of 546, or a mortality of 6.6 per cent. The percentages were : Maternity, 3.4 ; phthisis, 41.75 ; erysipelas, 1.28 ; Bright's disease, 15.5 ; pneumonia, 2.42.

Per capita, 34.7 cents ; drugs and liquors, 3.94 cents.

Homœopathic Hospital treated 5369 patients, with 273 deaths, or a mortality of 5 per cent.: Phthisis caused 50 per cent. of the deaths; pneumonia, 5.12 per cent. ; nephritis, 3.6 per cent.; erysipelas, 2.2 per cent.

The daily per capita was 31.67 cents ; drugs and liquors, .77 cents.

Leaving these figures for what they are worth, we desire to give a few from our report of 1886. During that year we treated 3733 patients, with a mortality of 7.5 per cent.; the highest, I think, in the history of the hospital. The previous year, 1885, we treated 3756 patients, with a death-rate of 6.9 per cent. There are no reasons which can be assigned for the higher mortality than the fact that a large number of patients carried through the months of the previous winter, died in the earlier months of the following year.

The 3733 cases were distributed as follows : Medical, 2104 ; surgical, 1239 ; venereal, 136 ; erysipelas, 119 ; ophthalmic, 70, and gynæcological, 65. Of this number, 1487 were discharged cured; 1399 improved; 176 unimproved; 279 died, leaving in the hospital on January 1st, 1887, 392. Phthisis caused 45 per cent. of the deaths; pneumonia, 7.8 per cent.; cardiac, 10 per cent.; nephritis, 2 per cent.; erysipelas, 84 per cent.

Our per capita was 29.38 cents ; drugs and liquors, .97 cents.

From September, 1875, to January, 1887, we have treated 1136 cases of erysipelas, with 31 deaths, or a mortality of 2.7 per cent. In connection with these figures, it should be stated that the large majority of our patients are the victims of intemperance; that of those who died, 6 were over fifty years of age; 1, five months; that 10 were only in the hospital four days, of which number 3 died within twenty-four hours after admission; that 1 was associated with typhoid fever; 11 with acute alcoholic delirium; 5 with chronic phthisis; 2 with acute pneumonia, and several with severe trauma.—*North American Journal of Homœopathy*, April, 1888.

The two city hospitals of Albany, New York, for the year ending September, 30, 1883 (see Report of Board of State Charities), reported: Homœopathic mortality, 5.33 per cent.; allopathic mortality, 7.26 per cent. In the Brooklyn hospitals, same year: Homœopathic mortality, 8 per cent.; allopathic mortality, 9.48 per cent. In the Buffalo hospitals, same year Homœopathic mortality, 5 per cent.; allopathic mortality, 14.73 per cent.

In the Denver, Colorado, hospitals, 1880, under allopathic treatment, 11.97 per cent; 1881, under homœopathic treatment, mortality, 7.34 per cent.; 1882, under allopathic treatment, mortality, 8.90 per cent.; 1883, under homœopathic treatment, mortality, 6.03 per cent.

The Figures from Private Practice.

About fourteen years ago, a well-known life insurance company of New York city conducted a series of examinations of the records in the health offices of several of our largest cities, with a view to ascertain the comparative number of deaths occurring in the practice of physicians of the two rival schools. These investigations embraced the records of Boston for two years, 1870 and 1871; of New York, for 1870, 1871, and 1872; of Philadelphia, for 1872; of Newark, New Jersey, for 1872, 1873; and of Brooklyn, for 1872 and 1873. These ten tables of statistics yield the following results, showing the average number of patients lost by each homœopathic and each allopathic physician in each of those cities:

					Allopathic losses.	Homœopathic losses.
Boston,						
1870,	.	.	.	.	. 17.76	10.05
1871,	.	.	.	.	. 14.76	8.25
1872,	.	.	.	.	. 19.63	8.26
New York,						
1870,	.	.	.	.	. 15.75	9.00
1871,	.	.	.	.	. 15.78	7.97
Philadelphia,						
1872,	.	.	.	.	. 19.03	12.87
Newark, N. J.,						
1872,	.	.	.	.	. 27.54	12.92
1873.	.	.	.	.	. 15.39	9.56
Brooklyn,						
1872,	.	.	.	.	. 24.08	11.62
1873,	.	.	.	.	. 21.56	9.95
General average,	.	.	.	.	. 17.88	10.02

1872 was the year of the terrific epidemic of smallpox in Philadelphia.

Thus we obtain the average losses by 4071 allopathic and 810 homœopathic physicians, reporting an aggregate of 80,918 deaths. The investigations have been so extensive, and the figures involved are so large, that no candid mind can refuse to accept their results as strikingly indicative of the vast superiority of homœopathic over allopathic methods of treatment.

RESULTS IN YELLOW FEVER.

We have drawn these statistics from far-off Germany, and from our Northern States and cities. The last table that we shall cite is obtained right here in your own Crescent City, after the terrible yellow-fever scourge had visited the lower Mississippi valley in 1878. A commission to investigate the subject and to report to Congress was appointed by the American Institute of Homœopathy. This Commission was composed of your own distinguished Dr. William H. Holcombe, as chairman, with the no less eminent Drs. F. H. Orme, of Atlanta ; L. H. Falligant, of Savannah ; J. P. Dake, of Nashville ; L. D. Morse, of Mem-

phis; T. J. Harper, of Vicksburg; W. J. Murrell, of Mobile; E.
H. Price, of Chattanooga; W. L. Breyfogle, of Louisville; T. S.
Verdi, of Washington; and B. W. James, of Philadelphia. A
body of more conscientious, upright, reliable, and skilful yellow-fever experts could not be got together in this or any other
country, and their testimony no man dares to impeach. This
Commission devoted a vast amount of labor to the examination
of health-office records, and the collection of information from
all possible sources, and they found that while homœopathic
physicians had lost in the various localities from 4 to 8 per cent.
and upwards, the allopathic loss was 13 to 18 per cent. In
Chattanooga, Tennessee, where the disease raged with peculiar
malignancy, the homœopathic loss reached the startling figure
of 36.4 per cent.; the allopathic mortality was 45 per cent.

WHERE ARE THE ALLOPATHIC FIGURES?

And now what need have we of further testimony of this
sort? If we could add table after table of statistics to those
already presented, it might, in some degree, corroborate this testimony, but it could not add either to their significance or to their
force.—"Tests at the Bedside," by Pemberton Dudley, M.D.

Homœopathic experiments at Zulezya, in Padolia, conducted
by Dr. Herrman, by order of his majesty, the Emperor of Rus-
sia. The experiments lasted one hundred days in the year 1829:
Received, 165; cured, 141; died, 6; remaining, 18. *Mortality*,
3.64 per cent. The 18 remaining suffered from incurable organic
defects, and had been treated without success in other hospitals
also.

At the Infantry Hospital at St. Petersburg, there were treated
by Dr. Herrman, in 1829–30, by order of the Emperor, 409;
cured, 370; relieved, 7; not cured, 4; died, 16; remained, 12.
Mortality, 3.92 per cent.

During the cholera in 1846, there were 242 patients treated
at the so-called Homœopathic Cholera Hospital, at Munich, of
whom only 6 died. After the cessation of the cholera, it was
determined to continue this as a homœopathic hospital, for
which the Chambers voted 4000 florins per annum. Consent

was refused to the Chambers, but hardly in consequence of the following ratio of mortality. The summary of cases treated from December 13, 1836, to the end of December, 1837, in this institution, in Munich, is as follows: Patients, 242; cured, 223; relieved, 13; died, 6. *Mortality*, 2.48 per cent.

Of 738 patients treated from 1833 to 1841, in the Homœopathic Hospital at Günz, 666 were cured; 10 relieved; 5 not cured; 29 died; received moribund, 17; remaining, 11. *Mortality*, 3.92.

In the Homœopathic Hospital at Gyöngyös, from 1838 to 1841, there were treated 271; cured, 219; relieved, 14; not cured, 7; died, 11; received moribund, 15; remaining, 5. *Mortality*, 4.06 per cent.

In the Homœopathic Hospital of the Sisters of Mercy at Vienna, from 1832 to 1841, there were treated 5161; cured, 4710; not cured, 89; died, 267; brought in moribund, 34; remaining, 61. *Mortality*, 5.02 per cent.

Summary of cases treated in Leipsic from 1833 to 1841: Cases, 4665; cured, 3984; relieved, 297; not cured, 127; died, 157; received moribund, 31; remaining, 69. *Mortality*, 3.57 per cent.

According to the above, the mortality of these homœopathic hospitals has an average of 4.22 per cent.

SUMMARY OF CASES IN VARIOUS ALLOPATHIC HOSPITALS.

Mary's Hospital in St. Petersburg in the year 1837: Patients, 3356; cured, 2261; died, 773; remained, 322. *Mortality*, 23.03 per cent. All Saints' Hospital in Breslau in the year 1833: Patients, 2443; cured, 1701; died, 409; relieved, 105; not cured, 60; remained, 168. *Mortality*, 16.74 per cent.

New York: Duration of Treatment Five Years (According to Dr. James Buckner).

Diseases.	HOMŒOPATHIC.		ALLOPATHIC.	
	Treated.	Died.	Treated.	Died.
Erysipelas	349	3	325	75
Diarrhœa	310	3	316	68
Fever without Typhus	3,273	41	1,994	107
Pleuritis	371	5	51	8
Small Pox and Varioloid	211	6	Accounts	Accounts
Scarlatina	102	3	Insufficient.	Insufficient.
Inflammation of Bowels	211	13	46	19
Fever of all kinds	5,399	334	4,367	487
Pneumonia	710	45	309	91
Dysentery	98	7	447	120
Typhus	2,126	293	2,373	380
Organic Diseases of Heart	109	17	56	29
Apoplexy	21	6	35	17
Phthisis Pulmonalis	502	194	247	120
Totals	13,792	970	10,566	1,521

Consequently the mortality here figures up in the homœopathic hospitals, 7.03, in the allopathic, 14.36 per cent.

Dr. Peters (John C. !) exclaims at this report: *Who, with such data before him, could be so great a fool as to subject himself to the heroic treatment of the old school?*

Charité Hospital, Berlin.

Year.	Patients.	Cured.	Died.	Mortality per cent.
1832	6,298	4,565	843	13.54
1833	6,749	4,966	909	13.46
1834	6,390	4.017	894	13.99
1835	6,323	4.499	715	11.31
1836	7,322	5,310	886	12.10
1837	8,214	6,010	1,039	12 61
1838	9,097	6,955	893	9.82
1839	10,616	8,277	1,052	9.91

St. James' Hospital in Leipsic in 1839: Patients, 1132; cured, 700; died, 117. *Mortality,* 10.33 per cent. In the wards of the general hospital in Vienna in the year 1838 there were: Patients,

20,545; died, 2678. *Mortality*, 13.03 per cent. In the year 1841 : Patients, 24,258; cured, 19,363; died, 3068. *Mortality*, 12.73 per cent.

The average mortality of these hospitals is 12.08 per cent. Thus, under homœopathic treatment, one patient in every twenty-three died, while under allopathic, one in every eight.

As regards the results of the treatment of *Cholera*, I will also give only the sums total from Dr. Rosenberg's work, where the details can be more fully seen. The summary of cholera cases treated *homœopathically* in different countries by different physicians, 14,014 patients; 12,748 cured; 1266 died. A *mortality* of 9 per cent.

Under allopathic treatment in various countries, 457,536 patients; 184,044 cured, and 222,342 died. A *mortality* of 48.39 per cent.

As regards the expenses, Dr. Rosenberg makes the following statement: In the year 1840 the cost for the daily support of a patient in the homœopathic stationary clinic at Leipsic was 3⅔ groschen [11 cts.]. During the same year the administration of general charity in Berlin set down the daily cost of one patient at 7½ groschen [22½ cts.]; thus in the Charité, the daily cost of a patient was about 3⅜ groschen [11½ cts.] more than in the homœopathic institutions.

Since, according to report, in the Charité about 10,000 patients are sustained, their support costs, if we assume as an average, that each patient remains twenty days in the hospitals, 62,500 thalers [$41,666.66⅔]. A like number of patients, remaining the same time under treatment in a homœopathic hospital, would cost per annum, 30,555 thalers, 13½ groschen [$20,370]. Hence the Charité, under homœopathic treatment, would save 31,945 thalers [$11,296] annually. We find the same proportions also in *Knolz's Darstellung der Humanitals and Heilenstallen* in Vienna for the year 1848, according to which a patient cost in these institutions about 17½ kreuzers more a day than in homœopathic hospitals, and that the government would have saved in these Vienna institutions alone 143,248 florins, 53 kreuzers, C. M. (Conventions Munze), had they been under homœopathic treatment. We now come to more recent dates.

Dr. Zessier was established in the St. Margaret's Hospital in Paris, and the opponents of homœopathy sought to expel either him or homœopathy. But they received from the administration of hospitals at Paris the following reply: "Before, as well as since the time of Hippocrates, physicians have always been of different opinions, and always will be. But we as managers of the hospitals must stand aloof from their schools, and we take no part at all in their contentions, which are more or less of a scientific character. We content ourselves merely with establishing the results, which each physician obtained in his service, as we do at present. In St. Margaret's Hospital we find two sections, one with 100 beds under Dr. Zessier, who treats his patients homœopathically; the other with 99 beds under Dr. Valleix, and after his resignation under Dr. Marotte, who treated their patients allopathically. The new-comers were put into the first vacant bed, whether it happened to be in one section or the other. Hence the test of two therapeutic methods occurred as much as possible under the same circumstances. The mortality now was as follows: In the years 1849, 1850 and 1851, there were treated in the allopathic section 3724 patients with 411 deaths, thus a mortality of 11 per cent.

"In the homœopathic section, 4663 patients were treated, with 339 deaths—a mortality of 8 per cent.

"Under such results we are far from meddling with the liberty of medical art, or from wishing to put any hindrance in the way of Dr. Zessier's treating his patients homœopathically; on the contrary, we would encourage him to persevere in his efforts *which can only benefit humanity.*"

In the same hospital, at the same time, the average duration of disease was twenty-three days in the homœopathic section; in the allopathic twenty-nine days, which thus, thanks to homœopathy, permitted, in a hospital of 100 beds, *aid to be administered to 300 more patients than* under allopathic treatment, or, in this manner, a hospital of 100 beds would be equal to an allopathic hospital of 120 beds. The cost of drugs under allopathic treatment, amounted to 23,522; in the homœopathic to two or three hundred, thus about the one-hundreth part.

Something similar happened at Thoissey, Department Aisne,

where Dr. Gastier managed the hospital of the place from 1832 to 1848. An allopathic physician at Máson, probably vexed thereat, declared in a political paper of the city, that the Board of Administration of this hospital had forbidden Dr. Gastier to practice homœopathy in this institution. Immediately thereafter the administation sent to the editor the following letter for publication:

"We cannot be silent under a perfectly groundless statement, which would presuppose us to mistake entirely the sphere of our duty and meddle with affairs entirely foreign thereto. The administration of the hospitals has been established for the purpose of controlling the possessions and revenues of our institutions, and to watch over their well being, as well as to see that each officer conscientiously discharges his duties, *but by no means to prescribe rules to the physician in the practice of his art*, for this field does not belong to our studies, and we. are strangers to it. It would, hence, have seemed ridiculous, if we had indulged ourselves in forbidding the physician of one hospital the use of any remedy which seems good to him. Medicine is a free art, and the manner of its exhibition must be perfectly free. Never, and this best proves the consideration which medicine enjoys, *never, at any time, in any land, have even absolute governments undertaken to prescribe or ?forbid this or that curative method to the physician.*

"We contradict the announcement of Dr. C. in every respect, since he has fallen into an error which is, to us, quite incomprehensible, but we also declare that, in case we had really the right which he ascribes to us, we should not be at all inclined to make use of it. Our register shows that, since the accession of Dr. Gastier, the *number of deaths, in proportion to the number of cases, has been much less than ever before; that the cost of medicine has been almost nil, and that the service has been sensibly relieved by simplicity and regularity.*"

Board of Administration.—Magot, Burgomaster, President; Challond, Adjunct; Lorin, Member of the General Council; Ducrest, Chaplain; Billand, Senior Director. GRAUVOGL.

CPSIA information can be obtained
at www.ICGtesting.com
Printed in the USA
BVHW011626220219
540828BV00029B/230/P